FITNESS BY LAWS

A UNIQUE SYSTEM TO WEIGHT LOSS FOR THE WOMEN OVER 40

JILL LAWS PT
Female fat loss coach

DISCLAIMER INFORMATION

Copyright 2023 by Jill Laws

All rights reserved.

No part of this publication may be reproduced, distributed or transmitted in any form or by any means, including photocopying, recording, or other electonic or mechanical methods, without the prior written permission of the publisher, except in the case of brief quotations embodied in critical reviews and certain oter noncommercial uses permitted by copyright law.

The author makes no guarantees to the results you'll achieve by reading this book. All business requires risk and hard work. The results and client case studies presented in this book represent results achieved working directly with the author. Your results may vary when undertaking any new business venture or marketing strategy.

TABLE OF CONTENTS

YOUR MINDSET MATTERS 1

THIS IS NOT A DIET! 3

STOP OVER COMPLICATING THINGS 5

LIFESTYLE 9

IT'S TIME TO LEVEL UP 9

ACTION 13

THE COMFORT ZONE IS THE DEAD ZONE 13

WEIGHT TRAINING 17

NOTHING BEATS THE FEELING OF BEING STRONG .. 17

SELF CARE/ ESTEEM / AWARE 23

BELIEVE ACHIEVE 23

PUTTING IT ALL TOGETHER 27

OBSTACLES AND CHALLENGES ALONG THE WAY 33

LETS RECAP 37

WHAT TO DO NEXT 47

ABOUT THE AUTHOR 49

This book is for any woman who struggles with weight gain
For any woman that has become a slave to the scales
For all the woman who have tried endless diets only to break them and feel deflated
For the woman who has lost her confidence and feels fed up of her reflection
For the woman who wants to gain back control,find balance and live her best life without spending hours in the gym.

> "I'm a much happier, stronger and more balanced version of myself, yes I put the effort in but I couldn't have done it without the support and passion of Jill. Thank you Jill. You have made me believe in myself again and I will be forever grateful for giving me my life back"
> -Jane-

JILL LAWS PT

Female fat loss coach

Chapter 1

Your mindset matters

Hey I'm Jill I have worked within the fitness industry coaching women for many years.

Having continually used this 4 point system and seeing the life changing results I've had with my clients, I felt I just had to share it with you.

I have worked with women just like you who are caught up in the constant diet trap and are a slave to the scales. Women who have tried endless fads, shakes and pills only to regain the weight they have lost and more.

I really hope you get some insight into how, by shifting your mindset, you can achieve the exact results you desire, and how you can change your body shape at any age. It's not as hard as you may think. I work with women every day and the key to weight loss is not found in cutting calories, it's found in establishing some healthy habits and ditching the yo-yo mentality diet culture.

> "Within two weeks of virtual training (I live in the Midlands and Jill in the South) I had found my mojo. Every symptom of the menopause had disappeared and the only way I can describe it is that I found myself. Yes, it's true 3-30 minutes workouts did all the above for me. The daily accountability really helped too"
> -Heidi-

Chapter 2

This is not a diet!

Our world is so fast paced and the current fitness industry is exploding with unrealistic claims as well as get ripped quick programs; from shakes to pills and potions. It's all out there.

I've been in this industry for over 20 years, working with women who want to gain control of their life and who are struggling to do so. We've all possibly been there; that awful photo or a reflection in the mirror and hating or feeling miserable with what we see. The clothes that just don't fit. That's enough for anyone to look up the latest trend or quick fix diet. The diet industry is estimated to be worth £60 billion per year and that's made up mostly of vulnerable women looking for a quick solution.

In this book I'm going to guide you through the four points of success that I use with myself and my clients. Now let's get this straight, this is not a diet book (diets have beginning and ends to them) and this is not a quick fix. What you're going to learn will actually be life changing. You will never have to diet again; you will gain confidence and feel more in control than ever before.

I wanted to write this book for every woman that's struggling and for every woman that just doesn't feel herself any more. I also wanted to write this book for every woman who is not living her best life because she lacks confidence, self belief and motivation to do anything about it.

It's time to step away from the diet culture and level up!

JILL LAWS PT

> "Jill has been instrumental in changing my attitude to fitness, and subsequently those changes are reflected in my health in the last 6 months. Jill takes on board that not everyone has the time to spend hours in the gym. She works you hard, encourages you and understands what you want to achieve and helps you get there. This lady knows her stuff'
> -Theresa-

Chapter 3

Stop over complicating things

In my opinion there's not a new shiny secret way to start your fitness and health journey (sorry if that disappoints you). I would actually say there's a "strip it all back and stop over complicating things" approach needed. Keep things simple. The industry has become so diluted with advice and it's just full of noise and confusion. You know, I was weight training a long long time ago and I still am. It wasn't fashionable like it is today, and every new influencer today is claiming they have found the hidden secret.

Well let me tell you now they really haven't. The body will always be the body. There's no secret! There's no new sexy exercise that's going to transform your physique in a few weeks. Your butt is your butt and the exercises that worked back then will still work now without the confusion.

Once you let go of the noise and the social media doom scrolling and start to understand the uncomplicated basics, you will be well on your way to success, and a much better balanced lifestyle; and guess what? It's not as hard as you think, it's not rocket science either and you can and will enjoy the process.

After my third child I really struggled to lose weight. I felt pretty low and my self esteem hit rock bottom, I started my journey like every other woman, bashing out calories in the cardio area, and guess what? It didn't work. I just kept thinking, 'eat less and run more!' That doesn't work either.

In fact that does more metabolic damage than good, hence the yoyo effect.

For anyone using that approach you will end up gaining more weight than when you started, as every time calories are dramatically reduced your metabolic rate is damaged; so then you end up in a repeated cycle for every holiday or wedding or social occasion. Hence the yo-yo effect.

You cut calories, look great for two weeks then it's back to your old self again because your eating plan is unsustainable. At the same time your weight is slowly creeping up as you're eating more and this usually happens on repeat throughout the year.

You can't keep starving yourself for a social occasion and it does not have a detrimental effect on your health in the long run.

I soon figured out that I was working really hard cutting calories and running for my life with no return, until I discovered, and introduced, weight training into my program.

Taddaaaa!

Suddenly my body changed, I never stepped on a running machine again and completely fell in love with the process. I could workout in half the time, eat more (100% win win) and my physique took on a completely new shape. Why had no one ever told me this before??

Once I had pulled on my big girl pants and started using the free weight area I wanted to spread the word to other women. I decided to gain all the relevant qualifications to do so. I wanted to learn everything there was to know. Unfortunately not many women listened. This was in the day and age of leotards and aerobics. But the obvious message to me was the women doing the aerobics had weight problems (go figure).

I've now been working with women for enough years in this industry to feel that I have earned my stripes and now I want to share the tried and tested fail proof system that I have always used for myself and with my clients, with amazing results.

FITNESS BY LAWS

You will never have to think about dieting again. We are going to banish the scales, and you will be able to change your body shape at ANY AGE.

You will learn the easy way, not only to lose weight but to keep it off for good without giving up the food you love or working out for hours on end.

I created my Fitness L.A.W.S. system, to help my clients achieve the results they desired and more importantly how to create a balanced lifestyle. Now I want to share this system with you and guide you through the process.

This 4 step system will cover how to upgrade your lifestyle, your mind and how to apply action even on the days you really don't want to. Learn how to fall in love with all aspects of weight training and how to elevate your self worth, confidence and step into your power. Not to mention how to change your body shape and tone all those wobbly bits.

Here are the four L.A.W.S that will be your ultimate key to success.

L - Lifestyle

A - Action

W - Weight Training

S - Self Care

I will cover each of these in more detail in the following chapters.
Then I will bring all of these elements together so that you can see how easy it will be to adapt the L.A.W.S. system into your everyday life.

JILL LAWS PT

> "Thank you so much for all your help, this has shown me I can get results in small bite size sessions without knackering myself. I feel so much stronger and a lot more toned. I'm really excited to see more results in the coming weeks."
>
> -sue-

Chapter 4

Lifestyle
It's time to level up

Are you ready to level up your lifestyle ?

When it comes to lifestyle, you have to let go of the all or nothing approach. This yo yo mentality is keeping you stuck. It's damaging your health and will never produce sustainable results or lifestyle change. I love to eat out and would never feel guilty about it. I love wine and can 100% polish off a bottle (not that I would suggest you do that) but I adjust and balance my calories and lifestyle to be enjoyable to me.

One bad day doesn't have to roll into a bad week or bad month; it's only when we give ourselves continuous restrictions does that tend to happen. Keep telling yourself you can't have cake, chips or wine and that's a sure fire way to be craving it all day every day.

Have you ever been on a diet that feels like a living hell and you're counting down the days till it's over?

Taking an 80/20 approach to your diet means you can have what you want, just in moderation. You don't need to only eat broccoli, fast or even turn vegan. If you feel you really want the cake just have it, just don't have the whole cake. Have enough to satisfy the craving then move on.

Let's also dismiss the fact there are bad foods. There are no bad foods, some just have more nutritional value than others.

For example a chicken breast has the same amount of calories as a doughnut, but it's going to fill you up a hell of a lot more and provide you with a great source of protein. So it will reduce your appetite and keep cravings at bay. Whereas a doughnut may result in a sugar crash and cause sweet cravings as well as not fill you up. So once you work out your daily/weekly calories, how you use them is really your choice, but banishing certain food groups because they are deemed bad is a recipe for disaster.

We all need to have a little of what we fancy, or enjoy a meal out with friends without guilt or restrictions. That's healthy, balanced living.

Once you start to apply this 80/20 rule, it will become so much easier to manage your day. If you have a day that maybe you feel you have over indulged or blown all your calories and then some, then just think about how you can do better tomorrow. It's not a big deal, and you haven't failed, you're just living your life your way and it's perfectly normal. You're human. I think this is where a lot of women fail, as we tend to beat ourselves up for falling off the wagon and that's when one day turns into one month.

"Oh I've blown it now so I may as well eat everything in sight"

No!

So let's completely forget about being on track or off track. You're now just going to be in that happy, satisfied middle.

When we fall into the world of fad diets and quick fixes it's true that you may reach your goals a lot quicker, but if you're starving yourself day in and day out you definitely won't keep the results because you're hungry, and miserable, and at some point you will have to eat more, because of hunger and cravings. so it's not sustainable long term. It's hell!

It's a quick fix, not a lifestyle and one you're usually willing and pleading to end.

Thinking more about your diet in moderation, will help you to achieve your goals and long lasting results, and you can still enjoy social occasions and the food you love.

Cheers to that !

FITNESS BY LAWS

Also as we examine your lifestyle, here's something I would like you to consider. Firstly, your daily activity. From walking the dog to cleaning the house; this all has a huge impact on our daily calorie consumption.

There's a term called NEAT, which stands for Non-Exercise-Activity-Thermogenesis. This term basically means the energy we use for everything we do, such as sleeping, standing, walking and housework etc. I always use a daily step count with my clients as walking is just so beneficial for clearing the mind, burning calories and it has a huge effect on weight loss.

In fact, walking has been shown to have loads of benefits. For example it reduces stress levels, lowers blood pressure, increases energy levels, improves sleep, helps with weight loss and costs nothing.

Hitting that step count everyday will make a big difference to your results and you will feel a lot more de-stressed and energized for it. It's so underrated.

So a top tip here would be to get a fit bit or some kind of tracker and start tracking your daily steps.

You will probably be very surprised with the results!

A good step count to aim for is around 10000 steps per day on average this is what I set for my clients on a daily basis.

To summarize

*No food will be off limits - there's no bad food

*You will apply an 80/20 rule - you will not starve yourself or cut calories too low

*Add more activity/steps to your day- You will track you steps and hit a daily step count of at least 10000 steps

JILL LAWS PT

> "I first found Jill on Facebook about a year ago. What she said about balance and consistency instead of punishing diets and exercise regimes to achieve results jumped out at me. I had the mindset of having to be skinny my whole life and so starved myself and exercised madly but then I would burn out and stop completely and so I would be fighting myself all the time. I have never been huge but not confident in myself and I wanted that. Jill has worked with me tirelessly over this year, through ailments which could have stopped me but with her encouragement and a few tweaks to my routine I have managed to stay on track. I feel I am now in a more balanced place and am feeling a lot more confident and as a bonus I now enjoy working out consistently rather than seeing it as a punishment to be endured all thanks to this lovely lady"
>
> -karen-

Chapter 5

Action
The comfort zone is the dead zone

Are you ready to take action? Are you ready to step out of your comfort zone ? Or are you waiting for good ol' motivation to appear ?

Motivation is a little bit of a myth really; we don't really jump out of bed and feel motivated (not even me). It's not really like that, and if motivation is something you're waiting for it could be a while before you do anything. Don't think you're broken because you lack motivation, you're normal, and it's perfectly ok. You just need to take a little action first. Action is always the way to go! Once you take action, motivation will follow so always take action first.

This leads us into the importance of planning, goal setting and habit change.

When adding a workout to your daily routine it needs to be short to start with. That's much easier to get your head around than planning for hours of working out. Always start small. It then needs to become a non negotiable activity, even on the days it feels hard. You have to take action.

It needs to become a habit, something you just do. So planning it into your day/week starts to form the change of behaviour you want to install into your lifestyle .

Maybe it's something you can schedule first thing in your day? You could set your alarm a bit earlier and just get it done. For me this works best. I like to get it done then get on with my day. It helps me think clearer and also have more energy and focus throughout the day.

I feel motivated once I've taken action and it definitely elevates my mood. But whatever time works for you, write it down and add it to your planner.

Results are the end product of consistency; consistency is definitely key here. Just showing up and taking action day in day out, even on the days you don't feel like it, will provide you with huge results and be a complete game changer.

When time is short, don't skip your session. Half a workout will always be better than no workout. This process is about building habits and going through the motions.

Schedule that workout into your day, get up earlier if need be but get it done whether you feel like it or not. Make it part of your day, just like brushing your teeth. Habits are much better formed by attaching them to something you already do, like an anchor. So attach that workout to your morning coffee or lunch break. Let it become just something you do, like a routine.

To make it more appealing try downloading something you want to listen to, a new podcast or a new playlist, something that will make you feel uplifted, and look forward to listening to.

You don't really need to rely on motivation, you just need a solid plan that is broken down into some small, easy, doable steps and that starts with action.

We can also take small productive steps forward by adding more water to our day. Adding more water to your day will really help with energy levels, digestion, kidney function and also it's great for your skin and overall weight loss.

FITNESS BY LAWS

I would also recommend adding more proteins to your lunches and evening meals. Adding more protein to your daily meals will help to stop cravings, aid with muscle growth plus keep you fuller for longer. This all helps with weight loss, hunger and cravings

Try also loading up your meals with extra veggies, experiment a little and add spices. Be adventurous.

All these small steps are easily done and will really add up over the coming weeks and months. Just implementing one or two things at a time will still make a huge difference

To summarize

- Plan your day- schedule your workout
- Think action first- motivation will follow
- Think small steps- big results-
- Look at how you can increase your protein intake
- Keep a water bottle with you at all times

> "I went to Jill because I can't be trusted on my own and nothing else has ever worked for me. From the start she has been amazing. She listens and genuinely cares about the people she works with and their goals. Jill has taught me SO much along the waySo I know why I'm doing things and how my body and the exercise I'm doing works. She's a genius.
> She's pushed me to achieve more than I ever thought I could do not just physically but mentally and we're only just getting started."
> -louise-

Chapter 6

Weight training
Nothing beats the feeling of being strong

Let's delve into the fun part, how weight training will change your mind body and attitude

First things first. I would like to list just some of the benefits of weight training for women but especially women of 40 plus years. This really is the time to do some kind of weight bearing exercise if you're not already.

Weight training has been proven to help with:

- Weight loss by increasing muscle mass
- Burn more calories at rest by raising the metabolism
- Protects joints by strengthening ligaments and tendons
- Increases Mobility/flexibility by using functional movements
- Balances hormones by stimulating the release of HGH (human growth hormone, which aids in building muscle and burning fat.
- Improves cardiovascular health by working the heart and lungs
- Improves mental health by releasing happy hormones
- Improves bone health by nudging bone forming cells into action
- Elevates mood by boosting endorphins and feel good hormones
- Boosts metabolism by increasing your resting metabolic rate. (RMR) Your RMR is the number of calories your body requires

to perform basic functions, digestion, breathing etc. This can be increased by the amount of lean muscle you add to your body.

- Improves posture by strengthening bones and muscles for better alignment and also core stability.

There are actually more things I could add, just ask our friend Alexa or google. The list goes on and on. So if weight training is so beneficial for women, why is it that when you walk into a gym, are you dumped on a cardio machine by the gym staff ? We are almost conditioned to feel as women that the weights are out of bounds! It's a crazy, very old fashioned attitude and no great surprise that so many women end up with zero results and feel miserable and deflated.

Now I'm not asking you to go all guns blazing! Quite the opposite in fact. If a gym feels a bit too much out of your comfort zone, then why not invest in some dumbbells for a home workout? This will work just as well to begin with and especially if you have children at home or a busy lifestyle.

When I started my own journey I just started small, no big lifts, just dumbbells and I took the time to learn some good technique. This is pretty important. Good form is key.

Another really important point is intensity. This is how hard you are working. A lot of women tend not to train with enough intensity and that's the most important ingredient for change. It's no good breezing through your workout without breaking a sweat. You need to be hot, the weights need to be heavy and the workout should make you breathless. If you're still chatting then think again my friend!

So skip the little dumbbells and stop fanny-arsing about with your workout! If you don't look like a sweaty mess that can't breathe then you're not working hard enough 😊 . Always remember you can take a break at any time, but you should not be pacing yourself.

FITNESS BY LAWS

Try using a scale of 1-10 to check how hard you are working, with 1 being way too easy (you could hit 20 reps) and 10 being too heavy (you can't do more than 4 reps) now work on a 7/8 intensity range.

Now you could possibly be thinking "oh but I don't want to bulk up. " This has to be one of the biggest myths on the planet! I can't tell you how many times I have heard this. Literally too many times.

So let's get this straight. You're not a guy!

Your testosterone levels (which is the hormone responsible for increasing muscle mass) are not high enough to end up bulky, so it's a complete myth. However you will be toned, feel stronger and you will change your body shape along with balancing out your hormones.

Now that's worth lifting a dumbbell for, isn't it?

Nothing beats the feeling of being strong.

When we talk about body image and body confidence, did you know that when you exercise, you release natural chemicals called endorphins? Endorphins trigger a positive feeling in the body which is why we feel so much better for actually getting it done. This will also improve self esteem and confidence.

Some studies show that people who exercise regularly benefit with a positive boost in mood and lower rate of depression.

As I mentioned before, the biggest game changer here is intensity. That's where the magic happens. Those last few reps that challenge you are the key. So say goodbye to the non results of pacing your workout, and say hello to the bad ass that's going to be working out with purpose.

Hell yeah!

To summarize

- Step out your comfort zone- that's the no results dead zone
- Workout with intensity- work between 7-8
- Think hot heavy breathless - sweaty mess
- Rest when you need to- Don't pace yourself

FITNESS BY LAWS

> I have been trained by Jill for quite some time now and my strength just keeps growing! She encourages and pushes me in the right direction. I love the accountability as this is a huge thing for me. I would recommend Jill to everyone.
> -Vicky-

Chapter 7

Self care/ esteem / aware
Believe achieve

As we enter our 40-50s and beyond, sometimes it can feel like a confusing uphill struggle. We naturally gain weight especially around our mid section. It's estimated that women between the ages of 45-55 gain at least half a kilo of weight each year. I think this tends to be the reason a lot of women go "to the eat less exercise more" scenario. During this time when our hormones change and decrease we become very stress reactive and insulin resistant due to a rise in cortisol.

Cortisol is a hormone more commonly known as our stress hormone. It's released by the adrenal glands, and has the effect of increasing the heart rate and your blood pressure. It's responsible for our fight or flight response, just in case there's a saber tooth tiger in aldi and you need to escape! This means that it prepares the body to either stay and fight the saber tooth tiger or to run away from it. Therefore it prepares us for short, intense exercise. Cortisol is also responsible for managing our metabolism, blood sugar and your sleep wake cycle.

Due to our changing bodies and a decrease of estrogen, your body will find itself in a frequently stressed state more often and therefore will produce more cortisol. If this is not addressed it will lead to weight gain especially round the middle/ waist area. Even though cortisol is vital to regulating your blood sugar levels by turning food into energy, excess cortisol can counteract the effects of insulin, causing insulin resistance, which can lead to weight gain.

So as you can see it's pretty important that along with the exercise we also reduce our stress levels in other ways too.

Stress management is super important and just as important as working out. We need to rest and recover. Adding walking to our weekly plan will reduce our cortisol levels (stress hormone) . Walking for weight loss is massively underrated. Take time to look after yourself, from a hot bath to a massage to a rest day. It's all going to have a huge benefit on your health.

Sleep is also a vital element and really important for our well being and keeps our cravings under control. Lack of sleep tends to lead us to craving carbs, biscuits and allsorts of sugary treats. Lack of sleep can cause our hunger-stimulating hormone ghrelin to increase which makes us crave more sweet sugary snacks.So aim for around 7 to 8 hours a night if possible, try to decrease screen time, reduce caffeine and food late at night, make sure your bedroom is not too hot and is a restful environment. Remove electronic devices, and try to create a relaxing bedtime routine.

When it comes to self care I also want you to look at other habits that may be holding you back or limiting your results or self belief. I want you to fully get your head in the game. The mind is a powerful machine, the driving force between what you want and what you believe you're capable of.

It's really easy to spend time on social media. We all do it but I want you to be aware of the limits you place on yourself and also how comparing yourself to others can be damaging to your health. When we start comparing ourselves to others it can have such a detrimental impact on our own self worth. It's so easy to think everyone has it all worked out, but we all have to start somewhere. No one gets to skip the beginning of any new journey, especially a health and fitness one, so don't compare yourself with someone that's been in the game a lot longer than you. We all have to start somewhere and have a day one. I did, and I was rubbish, a complete novice! But I soon learnt through my mistakes. The good news for you is that I have made these mistakes for you so you don't have to, and you now have this step by step guide.

FITNESS BY LAWS

You just need to start with some simple steps and take action. Maybe you have tried other fitness programs or diets countless times before that just haven't worked for you, so you're more than a little skeptical and I get that but be careful of the little voice in your head.

If you're already thinking this book won't work for you, then I hate to say it but it possibly won't, because you're already thinking about a failed outcome. But if you're excited about starting your journey then you're already halfway there.

You're already winning!

We believe all the stories we tell ourselves, whether they are good or bad. So change the narrative.

Believe achieve

To summarize

- Schedule rest and recovery days- to lower cortisol levels
- Walk to reduce stress levels- turn on fat burning
- Reduce screen/social media time- for better sleep
- Step away from the diet mentality- to avoid metabolic damage
- Listen to how you talk to yourself- be kind be positive
- Comparison is the thief of joy- don't do it.
- Celebrate every small win- You get what you celebrate

> Jill's advice and support is invaluable, she's pushed me to try things I never thought I could do and to succeed. She's always encouraging me to push on and reach higher and we always have a lot of fun doing it. She's given me so much confidence that I was really lacking. Thank you Jill for getting me to where I am now and actually enjoying going to the gym.
>
> -George-

Chapter 8

Putting it all together

So now we have a better understanding of all the elements for success.

How do we put all this into action?

LIFESTYLE

Let's take a look at what we will implement in lifestyle on a weekly basis
Read through and select 3 for your calendar (add notes page for own ideas)

1. Hit your step count + add extra protein to your meals
2. Hit your step count + add extra veggies to your meal
3. Hit your step count + take an extra bottle of water today
4. Hit your step count + extra walk with dog/kids/grandkids/random stranger
5. Hit your step count + Review your goals
6. Hit your step count + plan your meals for the week
7. Hit your step count + have dinner with friends without feeling guilty

Steps are a non negotiable so they will be in the daily calendar. So whether you're doing extra housework or walking the dog these will all add up. Our aim here is a minimum of 10000 per day or more

ACTION

Now let's have a look at the action steps that you will add to your calendar

Pick 3 off the list below (add notes page for own ideas)

1. You will not rely on motivation today you will take action
2. Download a podcast
3. Set your alarm an hour earlier to workout
4. Go to bed an hour earlier
5. Celebrate all the wins of the week
6. Find 2 motivating songs for your playlist
7. Plan your week ahead,

FITNESS BY LAWS

WEIGHT TRAINING

Now let's look at scheduling 3 workouts in your calendar per week. I've chosen Monday, Wednesday and Friday but you can choose the days that suit you.

Possibly start with a rest day in between as you become stronger and fitter you can add an extra day to exercise.

If you can't do 3, start with 2 and work your way up. This is your journey so work at your pace

Your training plan then may look like this

	Workout
Monday	Workout (never miss a monday) full body
Tuesday	
Wednesday	Workout/ weight training/ full body
Thursday	
Friday	Workout/ weight training/ full body
Saturday	
Sunday	

SELF-

Now let's look at SELF. Read the options below, and plan the chosen options into your calendar

1. Massage
2. Hot bath
3. Spa / self care treatment
4. Yoga / meditation
5. Limit screen time before bed
6. Limit social media time
7. Get an extra hours sleep

Choose 4 tasks from the self care table (add notes page for own ideas)

Once you have chosen from the table let's add them to your weekly planner.

Here's a sample of what your week could start to look like. With any new project it takes time to make it a habit, but planning ahead really helps.

I'm a great believer in starting small so if 3 or four items seems too much, make it a little smaller and just add 2 from the easier options. As long as you're moving forward you will always get results. It doesn't have to take over your life. Small steps in the right direction is the way to go.

FITNESS BY LAWS

Day	Lifestyle	Action	Weight training	Self
Monday	Walking	Download a new podcast	Workout 1	
Tuesday	Walking			Spa treatment
Wednesday	Walking	Get an extra hours sleep	Workout 2	
Thursday	Walking			Hot bath
Friday	Walking	Count your wins	Workout 3	
Saturday	Walking	Practice gratitude		Limit social media time
Sunday	Walking	Plan your week ahead		Limit screen time before bed

Try to change the options around per week to mix it up a bit. I always usually do my planning on a Sunday as it sets me up for the week. But when you do yours it is your choice. It will only take a short amount of time and you will add these around your normal day. Planning takes practice along with changing bad habits for good.

> Since working with Jill I have learnt new techniques and mindsets that have helped me tremendously with my fitness. I used to be a complete cardio bunny, never really touching heavy weights, to be honest I was unsure and nervous about what kind of exercises to do. Now I love weight training so much I have built a gym in my garage so I can keep progressing.
>
> -Jane-

Chapter 9

Obstacles and challenges along the way

So let's have a look at potential obstacles that can arise and throw you off track or that take you back into that self sabotage cycle.

Family commitment-you miss a workout - Tomorrow's another day get over it, plan your workout for the next day

Family celebration - you over indulge- have a stricter day tomorrow

Sick or ill health - you need time to recover- you need to rest.

Falling off track - you feel bad - start fresh the next day make a plan of action

Holiday / celebration -over indulge plus miss workouts- enjoy yourself with no guilt, you can still get your steps in.

As much as these things can blind side us, if you follow the simple 80/20 rule you can still win the day. The key here is not to give up. Do not let a bad day turn into a bad week or month. So no feeling bad about your decisions or circumstances ok? Just start each day with a fresh plan moving forward and look at areas you can improve as you go along.

So many of my clients have come to me stuck in a cycle of being good vs being bad and it's just a mindset shift that needs addressing. From this moment on you're not good or bad, you're just you and your choices will now be based on the outcome and goals you desire.

It may take a little longer than being strict with your nutrition but I can tell you it has 100% more chance of lasting and becoming a lifestyle with this new approach. And a lot more fun and a lot more sociable.

Come on, who wants to constantly eat out of plastic boxes? Chicken and broccoli can actually do one in my opinion 😊

Unless you're setting yourself up for a bikini contest then this is 100% not necessary, plus it's unsustainable for a long duration. So forget it. One thing I will add is that we pass so many of our habits and hangups to our children. They are always watching and it's paramount we set a good example to them.

It's important they understand that all food is ok in moderation, that there's no good or bad food and it's also to be enjoyed without guilt and restrictions. Now I'm not saying that take away or fast food is a good idea every night, but there's no harm once in a while at all.

Again moderation 80/20.

> I can not recommend Jill enough her positive attitude and passion inspire and motivates me to work harder to achieve my goals Jill encourages progress though a balance of support and challenge all delivered with a great sense of humor and the patience of a saint
> -Donna-

Chapter 10

Lets recap

So now you have all 4 bases covered let's have a quick recap.

You will now be operating on a 80/20 principle. Nothing is off limits when it comes to your nutrition but you are going to learn to be mindful of what you're consuming.

You're going to hit as many daily steps counts as you possibly can come rain or shine, even if it's in the house doing chores.

You're going to celebrate every win and use a planner to write down your goals, you will revisit your goals regularly and you will also plan your day and weeks.

This is a great habit to master but takes practice.

You will log what's working and what needs improving as you go along.

You will take time to rest and prioritize self care, you are worthy of looking after yourself.

You will add a strength training workout or 2 to your week,

Here's a sample of my week's planner now add your weekly actions into the planner.

JILL LAWS PT

MONTH: _____

WEEK: _____

MONDAY	TUESDAY
○	○
○	○
○	○
○	○

WEDNESDAY	THURSDAY
○	○
○	○
○	○
○	○

FRIDAY	SATURDAY
○	○
○	○
○	○
○	○

SUNDAY	NOTE
○	○
○	○
○	○
○	○

FITNESS BY LAWS

THIS WEEKS MAIN GOAL

-
-
-

WATER INTAKE

◊◊◊◊ ◊◊◊◊ ◊◊
   1L   2L   3L

WEATHER

TO DO LIST

-
-
-
-

NOTES

THIS WEEKS WINS

-
-
-
-

HOW WILL I IMPROVE NEXT WEEK

-
-
-
-

Now let's look at a sample workout. Everybody is different so one size doesn't always necessarily fit all but if we add a few basic exercises we can adjust them along the way.

This is a great place to start, focus on good technique and perfecting the movements. Once the exercises become easier it's time to add more weight or intensity.

Also remember the keys points you need to be
SWEATY
BREATHLESS
HOT

Work with intensity and concentrate on good form always.

Example workout 1

- SQUATS
- PUSH UPS
- BENT OVER ROW
- SHOULDER PRESS

4 sets of 4 exercises 8-10 reps but 10 should be your max

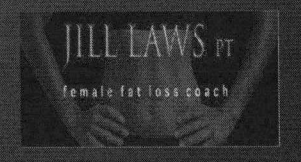

Example workout 2

- SQUAT & PRESS
- PUSH UPS
- WALKING LUNGE
- SHOULDER PRESS

4 sets of 4 exercises 8-10 reps but 10 should be your max

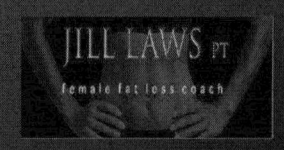

FITNESS BY LAWS

So there you have it, my four elements of success that have been tried and tested over and over.

You will never have to feel overwhelmed again with all the media misinformation out there.

You will never have to fork out a ridiculous amount of money on a new fad diet or shake.

You will never have to diet again or be a slave to the scales.

You will however be able to change your body shape and lose weight successfully without losing your mind.

FOR GOOD

Just implement the four actions below in simple small steps day by day.

Lifestyle-stepping away from damaging diet culture and finding a happy balance

Action-no more relying on motivation, just small daily actions

Weight training- Super short burst to speed up your metabolism and accelerate fat loss

Self- Lowering stress levels to help with weight loss and speed up results.

Before I sign off

and leave you with your planning. I wanted to tell you a little bit about me and what I do.

As I mentioned in the beginning, I entered the world of fitness and health to lose weight after my third child and I thank my lucky stars I fell into weight training or I would possibly still be overweight and on a treadmill now.

Fast forward to today I now have 4 children 7 grandchildren and at the moment 2 doggo's (I say at the moment as there's always room for more)

I exercise regularly for my mind as well as my health and body. It's a habit that's been formed out of routine; I get up, I get it done, then get on with my day. I really feel it has helped me tremendously during perimenopause and menopause on days when I felt I was possibly losing my mind.

A workout just resets my body and my focus and it will do that for you too, trust me. No one ever regrets working out.

This year my goal is to help as many women as I possibly can whether it be online in my private studio or by writing this book. It's a tough time and we need all the support we can get.

So many women lose their self confidence and I felt that too. Going into my 40's I really struggled but exercise helped me so much. I know it seems a hard thing to start if it's not something you have done before but just starting off super small with little steps can make a huge difference to how you feel and get you on that ladder to feeling so much better and stronger within yourself.

Most of my clients do not focus on weight loss, we focus on performance goals, like their first press up or pull up. This is much more fun, so much more rewarding and also shifts the weight loss mindset from the scales, as you have something a lot more fun to focus on.

Weight can fluctuate on a daily basis; from water to hormones, so weighing yourself day in and day out can turn a productive day into a miserable one. I ask my clients to take pictures and measurements only

FITNESS BY LAWS

to track their progress. This is the best way, better to be inches smaller even if you have gained a pound.

So get that tape measure out and use the next page to make a start on tracking your success today.

I believe in you

JILL LAWS PT

BODY MEASUREMENT CHART

DATE

1. bust

2. upper arm

3. waist

4. hip

5. thigh

weight

DATE

1. bust

2. upper arm

3. waist

4. hip

5. thigh

weight

DATE

1. bust

2. upper arm

3. waist

4. hip

5. thigh

weight

NOTES

© 2016 SPOTEBI • SPOTEBI.COM

Chapter 11

What to do next…

Now we have reached the end of this book, I sincerely hope that you have found it beneficial in more ways than one. So the next step for you is simple..

GET STARTED

Taking action is your next big step. Nothing will change if you don't take that step forward

You now have all the information you need to finally get the results you deserve without starving yourself or killing yourself with endless cardio workouts.

But if you're sitting on the fence or have any questions I would be more than happy to help you personally. You can email me and we can set up a free, no obligation strategy call. We can discuss your lifestyle, habits and nutrition to get you moving forward.

You can also work with me privately one to one online or in person. We all need our own cheerleader and I would love to be yours This is a great option if you feel you would like extra support and accountability.

Please feel free to email me on

jilllawspt@gmail.com

Also as we covered, adding protein to your meals is a really useful strategy to help stop those cravings, keep you on track. I have a handy protein guide that I send out to my clients. It explains all the benefits of protein in more depth and why it's so important. It also has some delicious recipes, if you would like a free copy just use the link below.

Protein guide

About the author

I'm passionate about getting real women just like you, results. I work with women everyday in my private studio and also online and I hear their everyday struggles, from trying every diet program under the sun to being burnt out and busy.

I also hear how confidence and self belief is so easy to lose as we age. But no woman should feel that they have to settle with being unhappy or not confident in their skin regardless of age and lifestyle.

I started my fitness career over 25 years ago mostly teaching group fitness classes and bootcamps. Once I discovered weight training I had to spread the word and knew this was the path I wanted to pursue.

After completing my Level 4 Personal Training qualification I also went on to study to become a Corrective Exercise Specialist, Back Pain Specialist, GP Referral, as well as Weight Loss Management and Nutrition.

All of these qualifications, as well as my experience helped me to develop unique programmes for women that had various challenges, backgrounds and goals. I made it my mission to create individual and unique programmes that helped women, rather than adopt a 'one size fits all' approach.

I love helping women achieve their goals and realizing their true potential. You can get the results you want at any age and even with a super busy lifestyle.

With consistency and support plus a little guidance and nudge in the right direction it's all 100% achievable.

Jill xx

Printed in Great Britain
by Amazon